Essential Oils

A Practical Guide for Beginners

By John Gordon

Table of Contents

Introduction

The use of essential oils dates back to several thousand years ago across cultures and civilizations for health, home and medicinal purposes.

History of essential oils is inseparable from the history of the science of medical herbs. Ancient Egyptians used aromatic plants for medical and cosmetic purpose, as well for the balm of their dead, 3000-3500 years before the new era.

Hippocrates, the father of medicine, lists numerous healing herbs in his writings.

In the 10th century, Arabic doctor Avicenna described in his writing over 800 herbs and their effect on the human body. He is mostly attributed to the development of the process of distillation of essential oils. From today's point of view, it is more likely that he didn't discover this process but perfected it, as archaeologists found primitive distillation devices which date back to the time before him.

In Europe, essential oils from Arabia became known sometime in the 12th century, and it's corresponds with starts and ends of Crusades in the Holy Land.

In the 16th century recipes for making vegetable oils and scents could be found.

In the 18th and 19th centuries, chemists investigated the active ingredients of medical herbs and identified numerous organic compounds (caffeine, quinine, morphine, atropine, etc.) which played a significant role, but the search for isolated agents nevertheless eventually turned to times of natural use of the whole plant. Essential oils where still in use, many remained in the official books of medicine and until the late 20th century, some of them, such as lavender, mint and some others, are used in pharmacy today.

Today, they are widely used in home cleaning products, beauty care items, aromatherapy and natural remedies.

Have you ever truly enjoyed the heady fragrance of rose or jasmine? If yes, you've experienced essential oils in some form. They are not just powerfully aromatic, but also beneficial. From the perspective of plants, these oils are responsible for their signature smell as well as protection and effective pollination.

So what exactly are these potently aromatic compounds? The compounds are tiny molecules that rapidly transform from an essentially solid or liquid state into gas at room temperature.

Have you ever tried opening a bottle of essential oil? If yes, you'll instantly be treated to a whiff of strong, pungent yet pleasing fragrance, even from afar. The aroma is immediately noticeable from a considerable distance owing to the chemical properties of these strongly aromatic compounds. The compounds spread through the air quickly and make their way into our olfactory glands.

This is why they are such a vital component of aromatherapy. These plants help keep the mind, body and spirit healthy.

Essential oils are fat free natural extracts from aromatic plants obtained by distillation, extraction or some other method of isolation. Different parts of the plant are used to obtain oil: flowers, dried buds, leaves, stems, grasses, wooden parts, bark, vegetable resins, seeds, fruits. Essential oils have a high penetration ability through the skin's surface layer, causing the lipophilicity of the molecule and lower molecular weight.

Because of its chemical structure, essential oil is already a perfume composition in itself, because it contains about one hundred different compounds - terpenes, alcohols, phenols, esters, aldehydes and ketones. To make the oil effective, it needs to be natural and pure.

What is lipophilicty?

Lipophilicity refers to the ability of the chemical compound to dissolve in fats, oil, lipids and non-polar solvents, such as hexanes or toluene. These non-polar solvents are lipophils themselves (in free translation: "fat-lovers"). Thus lipophilic substances tend to dissolve in other lipophilic substances, while the hydrophilic (water-loving) substances have a water-soluble and other hydrophilic matter.

Ancient Egyptians created essential oils by putting various plant parts in oil, and later straining it through thin linen.

Since these oils capture the real flavor, properties, and fragrance of the plant, they are referred to as its "essence." The unique and highly individualistic, aroma compounds give every essential oil its natural characteristic. Essential oils can either be extracted through the process of distillation or cold-pressing. When the oil is extracted, it is mixed with a neutral base carrier oil for making ready to use items.

Therapeutic plant oils shield the plant from insects and tough weather conditions. By utilizing essential oils, you are fundamentally leveraging the healing powers of nature. Essential oils comprise tiny molecules that can penetrate the body's cells to offer myriad benefits. Fatty oils that originate from larger molecules are unable to pass through the body's cells, which makes them non-therapeutic in nature.

The important factor that determines if a product is genuine essential oil is the process through which the oil is obtained. If it is extracted through alchemical process, the oils cease to qualify as authentic essential oils.

The goodness of essential oils originates from their anti-oxidant, anti-inflammatory, aroma and antimicrobial characteristics. One of the biggest reasons for their popularity and widespread use is the fact that they are natural healers that come with zero side effects.

Are you ready to know more about the planet's most tried and tested therapeutic mixtures? Do you want to know the benefits of these powerful compounds and how they can be included in your everyday living? Do you want to know how you can create your own essential oils?

More than 3,000 different types of aromatic compounds are classified to date, each varying in nature and properties. Features differ from one plant type to another, and within the same botanical type.

The unique ratio of components present in the aromatic compounds is what differentiates them and awards their individual virtues. For pure essential oils, the composition can change depending on multiple factors, including weather, location, method of preparation, distillation duration, growing year and season.

Essential oils have many uses and benefits, the most common being aromatherapy. In aromatherapy, the oils are either taken in through the inhalation process or gently massaged into the skin. Ingestion isn't always recommended since it is generally unsafe or harmful for health. The chemicals present in all essential oils influence our body in different ways depending on their unique characteristics and properties.

When some oils are inhaled, their individual properties are believed to have an impact on our physical, psychological and spiritual conditions. Through massage, the chemicals can be completely absorbed by the skin.

Inhalation of essential oil fragrances is known to trigger specific limbic system areas, which play a significant role in one's emotions, feelings, behavior, smell and memory. Did you know that our limbic system, in fact, plays a huge role in storing memories?

This will explain why you associate certain smells with specific feelings, memories or experiences. The limbic system is also responsible for affecting our unconscious psychological functions, including heart rate and blood pressure.

All these factors go on to determine the overall oil essence and grade. One of the best parts about essential oils is that it can be used as a standalone or in complex oil blends based on the specific benefit users seek.

Today, people from several cultures, including Japan are incorporating the use of essential oils into their everyday life. In fact, in Japan, these natural beauties have made their work into the workplace as well. Essential oils are ingeniously employed in Japanese workplaces to help employees stay focused, efficient and eliminate errors. Some corporations in Tokyo have installed air-conditioners that emit a variety of fragrances throughout the day to keep workers energized, alert and invigorated. For instance, it's lemon early in the morning to awaken their senses and prepare them for a long day at work. By mid-morning, the fragrance changes to rose, followed by cypress in the afternoon. Many corporations use peppermint, lemon, and lavender for creating a positive, upbeat and inspiring atmosphere. The essential oils are often used according to the time of the day, and the therapeutic value they can add at that particular time of the day.

Chapter One: Health Benefits of Essential Oils

Though essential oils are said to possess multiple benefits, not much is known about its impact on physical health by the average person who relies more on chemical based solutions, pills, cosmetics and inorganic mixtures for their everyday needs. Here are some health benefits of essential oil.

Elimination of Stress and Anxiety

Spread a few drops of lavender oil throughout your home or room for decreasing feelings related to stress, anxiety and tension.

Research has pointed to the fact that around one third of Americans use some type of complementing or alternative therapy for helping them manage their discomfort causing condition more effectively (Barnes, et al. 2004). Many studies reveal the strong fragrance of essential oils work as therapy to offer relief from tension and anxiety. Massage using essential oils for relief from anxiety, stress and tension.

Insomnia and Sleep

Inhaling lavender oil has a potently positive effect on the quality of sleep and sleep patterns. Sprinkle a few drops of lavender essential oils on the pillow (you can also add a few drops of Chamomile). Alternatively, keep a cotton ball with a few drops of both the oils added to it and place it near you while sleeping. The inhalations will penetrate deep into the body to award you a more peaceful and relaxed sleep.

You can also have a few drops of lavender oil to a carrier oil, and gently use it for massaging your back just before going to bed for sound, anxiety-free sleep.

Antibacterial Infections

Essential oils are known for their anti-bacterial and anti-microbial properties that can combat bacterial ailments and infections. Peppermint and tea tree oil have been tested multiple times for their anti-bacterial characteristics. A few drops of these essential oils can help keep a place free of bacteria and harmful microbes.

Migraines and Persistent Headaches

Dabbing a few drops of peppermint oil in ethanol and rubbing it on the forehead and temples of a person is said to reduce persistent headache and migraine. One can also get effective relief from headaches by massaging the skin with lavender or peppermint oil. Using a mixture of sesame oil and the chamomile essential oil on the forehead or temples is believed to be an effective treatment for migraine.

Persistent headaches may be effectively treated by adding a couple of drops of lavender, eucalyptus and peppermint essential oil with per 6-7 drops of regular carrier oil. Gently massage the mixture on the temples and all over the forehead for instant relief from headache.

Relief Against Common Cold and Flu

Oregano oil is a known flu fighter, which is said to possess natural antibacterial characteristics. It is also effective for combating colds and a general feeling of sickness. Another extremely potent treatment for the common cold is adding a few drops of eucalyptus oil on a kerchief and sniffing it continuously. Eucalyptus is also effective for other respiratory issues such as sinus, bronchitis and persistent allergies. It is also known to cleanse the body from toxins.

Nausea, Chest and Sinus Congestion

Peppermint essential oil when rubbed on the soles of the feet is an excellent home remedy for nausea and mild fever. It can also be added to cleaners and home-made soaps for more effectiveness against sinus congestion. If you're suffering from persistent chest congestion, add a couple of peppermint drops or other essential oils in a diffuser or steaming water, and breathe deeply into the pot for clearing the sinus.

Eliminating Bodily Toxins

Black pepper essential oil is one of the best natural solutions for eliminating harmful toxins from the body. It also facilitates digestion, induces perspiration and removes uric acid from the body. Traces of gases in the intestines are removed, and not allowed to grow with regular usage of black pepper essential oil. It is also known to be effective against arthritis, spasms and rheumatism. Black pepper oil cuts down the growth of bacteria, battles premature aging and fights radicals that can cause harm to our body in several ways.

Improves Blood Circulation

Some essential oils such as cinnamon facilitate blood circulation and are excellent for combating blood impurities, wounds, healing, relief from pain, menstrual cramps, skin infections and issues related to blood circulation.

Here's a list of essential oils that are beneficial for your health

1. Chamomile Essential Oil

Chamomile has multiple health benefits and can be an effective remedy for almost every health issue since it is known for its antiseptic, antiphlogistic, antibiotic, antineuralgic, anti-inflammatory, analgesic, digestive, anti-infectious, antidepressant (phew!) and several other properties.

Chamomile essential oil has several benefits, including being an effective treatment for spasms and wounds. It prevents wounds from becoming infected. The versatile essential oil is also a super effective depression fighter and mood enhancer. It also helps fight neuralgic pain by lowering swelling in the affected blood vessels.

Looking for relief from inflammation and fever? There's chamomile essential oil to the rescue. It helps get rid of waste gases, facilitates bile discharge, fights inflammation arising from fever, heals pain, decreases fever, and is known to be extremely beneficial for our liver. Chamomile oil also helps in enhancing the function of our nervous system, lowering spasms, killing germs, facilitating better digestion, and fighting bacterial infections to give you glowing health.

No wonder it is one of the most popular arsenals in many natural medicine boxes across the world.

2. Frankincense Essential Oil

Frankincense essential oil is another very popular essential oil that offers tons of health benefits. It is known to be an effective antiseptic, astringent, sedative, digestive, tonic and much more. Frankincense essential oil offers protection against wounds turning infectious. It is also effective for scar healing and keeping the body's cells healthy. Frankincense aids digestion balances, menstrual cycles, helps in curing cough and cold, soothes inflammation, reduces anxiety and offers you glowing, overall health.

3. Helichrysum Essential Oil

Helichrysum essential oil is known for its antispasmodic, anti-inflammatory, antimicrobial, antiphlogistic, fungicidal, anticoagulant and other properties. Patients are advised to use this particular essential oil because of its healing and remedial benefits. Helichrysum essential oil is known to decrease spasms, fight allergies, maintain blood fluidity, reduce microbial infections, clearing clots, decreasing inflammation and preserve the health of our nervous system.

Furthermore, it decreases different kinds of inflammatory conditions, reduces cough, clears the lung passageway of phlegm, heals wounds and scars, ensures skin health and fights bacterial infection. Helichrysum essential oil is said to be exceptionally good for the liver while facilitating regeneration of the body's cells.

4. Marjoram Essential Oil

Marjoram essential oil is antispasmodic, antiviral, digestive, laxative, diuretic, expectorant and much more.

Marjoram essential oil decreases pain, cures spasms and offers relief from cramps. It also offers protection against wounds, impedes the growth of virus and bacteria, removes additional wasteful gases from our intestines, offers relief from headaches, facilitates perspiration (for helping the body get rid of toxins), aids smooth digestion, clears menses, offers relief from common cold and cough. Marjoram is a known bacteria and fungus killer, blood pressure reducer, constipation curer and nervous system soother. It is known to ensure the overall health of your digestive system and stomach.

5. Peppermint Essential Oil

Peppermint essential oil is utilized as an anesthetic, antispasmodic, expectorant, stimulant, astringent, decongestant, hepatic, carminative, stomachic, cordial, cholagogue, nervine and much more.

Peppermint essential oil is a staple in several medicine boxes owing to its pain relief and relaxing properties. It is widely used for offering relief from pain, reducing spasms, strengthening gums, preventing hair loss and skin lifting purposes. It is also effective in facilitating muscle firmness, boosting memory and brain functions, facilitating bile discharge, clearing chest congestion, and promoting breathing.

Further, peppermint oil offers menstrual support, decreases fever, is said to be exceptionally good for the liver, facilitates perspiration and contracts blood vessels. It also helps the breathing pathway expel phlegm.

6. Rose Essential Oil

Rose oil has been utilized as an antidepressant, antiseptic, antiviral, astringent, hepatic, nervine, laxative, stomachic and more. Traditionally, it is a mood booster and depression fighter. Rose essential oil is also believed to offer relief from spasms, viral and bacterial infections and sexual disorders. It is known to be a natural libido enhancer and muscle tightener. Rose oil is believed to be effective in combating hemorrhaging.

Furthermore, it stops bacterial growth, facilities secretions of digestive juices, heals wounds and scars, helps in purifying the blood, enhances liver health, fights nervous system disorders, offers relief against constipation, and is great for overall stomach health.

Chapter Two: 60 Power-Packed Uses of Essential Oils in Daily Life

With its antioxidant, anti-inflammatory and anti-bacterial properties, it's little surprise that the healing oils can be resourcefully used for multiple purposes including health, home and beauty. Are you prepared to experience the bountiful benefits of essential oils? Here are 60 power-packed benefits and uses of essential oils.

Home and Everyday Living Uses

1. Natural insect repellent – Essential oils such as lemongrass oil and eucalyptus oil can be combined with coconut oil to create natural insect repellents or sprays. The mixture can be applied on the skin to keep mosquitoes away or used as a spray.

Certain oils, including citronella, have a significant effect on certain kinds of mosquitoes for about a couple of hours. When used with vanillin, it offers protection for up to 2-3 hours from mosquitoes.

2. Air cleaner – Cinnamon oil sprayed all over the home or garden can clean the air of microbes, and make it purer for breathing. Use a diffuser for circulating the essential oil within your space. Sometimes the air around the house starts smelling stale. Simply add a few drops of your favorite essential oil to water and use it in a spray bottle. Shake it well, and simply spread around the house. What are the best essential oils for air freshening? Pine and Fir (the silver variety) can work well. They infuse the freshness verdant green forests and clean mountain air in your home to lend it a nice nature-based touch. Want to make the fragrance even more attractive? Add a few drops of lemon to the mix.

3. Aromatic home – Your guests will be awed at how wonderful your home smells if you diffuse a few drops of orange and clove essential oils (add a hint of rosemary too) all over the place.

4. Garbage can freshener – Add a few drops of tree or lemon essential oil in the trashcan to minimize the stale odor and kill microbes.

5. Fresh produce wash – Washing fresh produce with a couple of lemon essential oil drops makes them cleaner.

6. Vacuum cleaner – Add a few drops of your preferred essential oil in the vacuum cleaner bag for giving the home a refreshing fragrance while cleaning.

7. Burnt pots and pans cleaner – Add a couple of lemon essential oil drops to boiling water for getting rid of stubborn burnt food that does not go with regular washing methods.

8. Mint tea – Fancy a cup of refreshing mint tea after a tiring day? Add a couple of peppermint oil drops to any cup of tea to lend it a nice, refreshing, minty flavor.

9. Smoke reducer – Add a few rosemary essential oil drops (or tea tree/eucalyptus oil) in a bottle and diffuse around the house to eliminate cigarette smoke.

10. Multi-purpose home cleaner – Combine four drops each of tea tree and lemon essential oil with warm water for using as a natural, multi-purpose cleaner, especially for countertops and other kitchen surfaces.

11. Refrigerator purifier – To purify the fridge while cleaning, combine a few drops of grapefruit or lime essential oil with the warm rising water to purify and freshen your fridge.

12. Natural sunscreen – Combine coconut oil, shea butter and lavender oil, which can be stored in a bottle to make for an excellent chemical-free sunscreen.

13. Clean smelling kitchen – Mix a couple drops of citrus or clove oil into a pan of boiling water to eliminate overpowering cooking smells. When you are cooking something that emits a rather overpowering odor, neutralize it by putting a pan of water on the gas until it starts boiling. Add a few drops of cinnamon or clove to the water. The aroma emitting from these spices will mask the strong, pungent odors originating from your cooking. Keep essential oils such as cinnamon and clove handy in the kitchen for multiple creative uses.

14. Unique baby shower gift – Give the soon-to-be-parents and the baby a wall diffuser, infused with calming and soothing lavender essential oil.

15. Bathroom freshener – Add a few drops of lemon essential oil on a cotton ball and leave it in the toilet for afresh smelling bathroom.

16. Clean utensils – Want fancy sparkling, clean utensils? Add a couple of lemon oil drops in the dishwasher for spotless, clean utensils.

17. Shower scum remover – Combine four drops of eucalyptus oil with four drops of tea tree oil and lukewarm water. Put the mixture in a spray can and use it in the shower as a natural mold killer. There! Who said essential oils were only about health and aromatherapy?

18. Carpet cleaner – Want a natural and fairly inexpensive carpet cleaner? Combine Borax with around 10-15 drops of tea tree for an effective carpet cleaner. A stale carpet smell can be eliminated by adding a few drops of essential oil (10-12 drops) to around 200 grams of cornstarch. Mix it well, and keep in a container for

a day or two. Shake it well before using and spread it on your carpets for a few hours. Later, hoover it and, boom, you have the freshest smelling and cleanest looking carpets!

19. Holiday scent – It's Christmas and you want something that spreads a wonderful holiday fragrance to remind you of the festivities. Combine a drop of sandalwood, pine and cedarwood oil on the fire log for around half an hour before burning logs.

20. Bridal shower gift – Want to make a quick and effective bridal shower gift? Here's how you can make the ultimate romance potion. Combine 15-20 drops of sandalwood essential oil with a few drops (4-5) of cocoa, rose and vanilla each to a neutral lotion. The results will be nothing short of stunning.

21. Eliminate stinky shoe odor – Yes, we've all dealt with persistent and repulsive shoes. A great tip for eliminating a strong shoe odor is to combine some tea tree oil drops with lemon drops and leave it in the shoes for a while.

22. Glowing skin – If you are after healthy, glowing skin, combine a few drops of rose essential oil to your favorite face moisturizer. It is one of the world's priciest essential oils.

23. Natural aphrodisiac – Sandalwood is a natural aphrodisiac that is believed to enhance the libido and improve overall sexual energy.

24. Boost metabolism – A few drops of grapefruit oil can be added to water and consumed internally to help boost metabolism

25. Multiple uses with rosemary – Rosemary is a natural, chemical-free homemade hair thickener that can be added to just about any natural shampoo to act as a natural thickening agent. The essential oil is also great for enhancing memory and

cognitive functions, thus it's great if used while working or studying.

26. Eliminate pet odor – Mix around ten to fifteen drops of lavender essential oil in a tiny spray bottle containing apple cider vinegar. Mix it well, before spraying around the house for getting rid of stubborn pet odor.

Lemongrass is great for eliminating unwanted pet odor. Add around 10-12 drops of this essential oil to half a bucket of warm water (and daily cleanser), and simply mop the area where pet odors are really strong. Lemongrass or any preferred essential oil will leave your space smelling fresh, bright, and positive. The pets will end up happy too!

27. Aroma candles – Add some drops of your favorite essential oil fragrance to melted wax while it's hot, and the candle has been burnt for a couple of minutes. The space will be lit up with a pleasant, fragrant smell.

28. Fragrant cards – want to spread more holiday cheer with your Christmas greeting cards or letters? Essential oils are to the rescue yet again! Scent your cards with essential oils to lend them a special, fragrant holiday touch.

29. Fragrant bath towels and napkins – Scent your daily use napkins and bath towels by sprinkling a few drops of your preferred essential oil on a tiny piece of cloth and throw it with the towels and napkins. You can also add a nice fragrance to your clothes by adding a few drops of your preferred essential oil into the dryer. Add a couple drops of the oil to a tiny cloth and release it into the dryer with your clothes. Pick something light and floral. You do not want something that's overpowering because strong smells will linger. Any floral or citrus based oils should work well in this case. Just ensure the smell is not too strong.

30. Scented air-conditioned air – Want fresher smelling air-conditioned air? Place a cotton ball with your favorite essential oil in front of the air-conditioner vent for fresher and cleaner smelling air.

31. Spider repellent – Spray a few drops of peppermint essential oil combined with water near your doors, windows and the entrance porch. You can also add a few drops of peppermint essential oil and leave it in window and door corners to repel spiders from entering through any available opening. Utilize similar methods for rodents and other creatures that make their way into your home.

32. Bring artificial flowers to life – You can bring artificial flowers to life by combining a few drops of floral essential oil with water and spraying it on flowers. Shake the mixture in the sprayer before use and refill as needed. This makes your silk flowers appear more real and fragrant.

33. Creative projects – You can make cut-outs of trees, such as pine, from paperboard. Glue green paper on it to give it a nice, realistic appearance. Now spray a few drops of pine essential oil on it to lend it a fragrant pine feel. This resourceful tip can also be used during Christmas to add to the festival cheer.

34. Natural cooking flavors – Want to add natural and delicious flavors to your cooking? It's essential oils to the rescue again. Though the consumption of most essential oils isn't recommended, some varieties like lime and peppermint can be used in edible items, and in fact, lend it a brilliant flavor and aroma. Their vivid, rich aromas can kick in a nice flavor even into a boring looking meal. For instance, add a couple lime drops to salsa or your own marinade for making grilled fish. Make your hot cocoa even more lip-smacking by adding a few drops of peppermint. It can also be added to a freshly made pasta sauce. There's just no stopping how creative you can get with essential

oils in the kitchen. Just ensure the oils are safe for consumption and used in the right quantity. Generally, peppermint, nutmeg, basil and lemon are popular for cooking.

35. Scented underwear drawers – Add a few drops of your favorite essential oil on a cotton ball and place it inside your underwear drawer for fresh smelling undergarments. Each time you open the drawer, you will be treated to a nice, light, flirty, sensual fragrance that will capture your senses. You can use any exotic and sensual smelling essential oil such as rose, lavender, ylang-ylang or jasmine. The garments will also absorb the strong fragrance of these essential oils and help them smell ravishingly good.

Similarly, to have a fresher smelling wardrobe, mix 2-3 drops of lavender or basil essential oils on a ball of cotton wool. You will be welcomed by an inviting and fresh spring aroma in your wardrobe.

36. Bacteria-free skin – Do you have pesky, persistent pimples that do not go away? Essential oils have got you covered there too. Throw away harsh, chemical-ladenanti-acne creams, and show your skin some natural love by opting for tea tree oil. It naturally kills bacteria and germs responsible for the spread of acne. It is also effective against dandruff, fungus in nails and bug bites. Another beneficial anti-acne agent is thyme.

37. Natural hair conditioner – Parched, dry and fuzzy hair is best treated with a dose of natural oil instead of chemical-infused conditioners. Pick a solid moisturizing essential oil like argan oil that includes fatty acids and vitamins. Castor oil is another effective natural conditioning agent.

38. Natural skin brightener – Do not let dull skin hold you down. Keep your face shining bright and beautiful with a dash of jasmine or rose essential oil to your beauty arsenal. Rosehip oil is

generously laden with lycopene, which is a known skin rejuvenating agent. Jasmine helps keep the skin supple and reduces stretch marks.

39. Anti-aging treatment – Forget spending thousands of dollars on expensive and worthless anti-aging creams that only end up frustrating you due to lack of results. Instead opt for essential oils such as frankincense and geranium. Geranium essential oil is packed with astringents that keep the keep the skin tight and facilitate the creation of new skin cells. Frankincense also possesses anti-aging results, while also helping control oiliness and dermatitis.

40. Natural exfoliation – Want a natural remedy for glowing, fresh and youthful looking skin? Exfoliation is the key. Remove dead cells naturally to make way for renewed skin. Essential oils are also effective for evening out the skin tone and lightening dark spots (or tanning) for a more flawless look.

41. More natural sunscreen – Vitamin A and beta-carotene found in carrot seed oil are helpful for skin detoxification and cell growth. It also helps protect the skin from harmful elements in the environment. Carrot seed oil is also known to be an excellent natural sunscreen.

42. Fight cellulite – Want a quick and effective remedy for stubborn cellulite? Simply mix 5-6 drops of grapefruit essential oil with around 2 teaspoons of carrier oil (coconut oil should be fine) and gently rub on the cellulite region.

43. Perfumes – If you want to smell good without investing in heavy, chemical-laden fragrances, opt for fresh, natural smells such as lavender. Just dab a few drops of vanilla, jasmine or lavender on your wrist, and you'll be good to go for the next few hours. For men's colognes, work with clove, sandalwood or

cypress. You'll be amazed by how fresh, long-lasting and natural these fragrances will be.

44. Acne treatment – For getting rid of acne naturally, make a natural, home-based face wash by combining honey (the rawer it is, the better) and tea tree oil. Rub the mixture gently on your face for a couple of minutes. Rinse with cold water. Tea tree oil fights skin bacteria (that causes acne and other skin conditions) to give you even and healthy-looking skin.

45. Natural toothpaste – Mix some sea salt, coconut oil, xylitol and baking soda with a few drops of peppermint essential oil for making your own fresh-smelling toothpaste.

46. Stronger nails – Combine 10 drops of myrrh, lemon, and frankincense essential oils with a couple tablespoons of Vitamin E oil. Rub this mixture on the cuticles regularly for stronger and healthier nails.

47. Natural teeth whitener – Mix lemon essential oil, strawberries (the fresher, the better) and coconut oil. Apply the mixture to your teeth and rub gently for about 2-3 minute. Rinse.

48. Natural wrinkle reducer – Try this blend. Combine 3-4 drops of sandalwood, frankincense and geranium essential oils with a neutral lotion and apply the mixture all over your face, while avoiding the eyes.

49. Reduce dandruff – Mix 4-5 drops of lavender and rosemary essential oils with two to three tablespoons of neutral oil. Massage the mixture thoroughly on the scalp. Leave for 15 minutes. Shampoo your hair to get rid of the mixture. Apply regularly, and you'll notice a visible reduction in the amount of hair dandruff.

50. Natural sole crack remedy – Combine 3 drops of lavender essential oil with 2 tablespoons of carrier oil (preferably

coconut). Gently rub in on the cracked area before going to bed. Do not forget to put on a pair of socks to keep the area covered.

51. Cure nausea – Inhale peppermint oil a few times to reduce a compelling feeling of nausea. A few drops of the oil can also be applied to the chest and neck region for combating symptoms of nausea. Ginger is another much sought after essential oil when it comes to reducing nausea.

52. Hangover relief – Combine six drops each of lavender, cedarwood, rosemary, grapefruit, lemon and juniper essential oils into a relaxing warm bath to enjoy relief from uncomfortable hangover symptoms. These oils will make you feel instantly energized and rejuvenated.

53. Manage appetite – Essential oils can act as a natural appetite curbing agent. Take a few whiffs of cinnamon and peppermint essential oils to curb your appetite and regulate the body's blood sugar level.

54. Natural lice treatment – Head lice playing havoc with your hair? Mix 4 drops of lavender, eucalyptus and thyme essential oils with neutral smelling oil. Apply the mixture evenly throughout the scalp. Leave for about 30-40 minutes with a shower cap on the head. Shampoo to rise off the solution. Use this remedy periodically, and the lice will be gone.

55. Natural weight loss – Mix cinnamon, grapefruit and ginger essential oil and consume this natural supplement thrice a day for boosting the body's metabolism. However, consult with a medical practitioner first before using any supplements to know if they are compatible with your health and physical conditions.

56. Soothe sunburns – Mix lavender essential oil with a tablespoon of carrier oil. Apply the mixture gently on the skin using a cotton ball.

57. Relief from morning sickness – Yes morning sickness caused by pregnancy can be terrible. But like everything else, essential oils have got a solution (well, literally!) for this too. Add 2-3 drops of lemon, orange and ginger on a handkerchief, and inhale for quick relief against pregnancy-induced morning sickness.

58. Decrease back pain – Combine ginger, cypress and peppermint essential oils with carrier oil for a nice and natural back and neck pain reducing rub.

59. Treat bruises naturally – Make a hot compress from essential oils to treat bruises naturally. Simply add 6 drops of lavender and frankincense to around 5 ounces of warm water. Soak completely. Apply this mixture on the bruised area.

60. Natural deep conditioner – Mix 16 drops of rosewood essential oil with 6 drops each of lavender and sandalwood essential oils. Add the mixture to carrier oil. Now, place the entire mixture into a tiny plastic bag dipped into warm water for heating it up. Apply generously throughout the hair and wrap for about 25 minutes. Rinse off with a shampoo.

Chapter Three: Aromatherapy

What is Aromatherapy?

Aromatherapy is a treatment that is now wildly used in the field of holistic therapy at massage centers, luxury spas, hospices, yoga studios and chiropractic centers. So what exactly is aromatherapy?

Aromatherapy is using essential oils extracted from various plants for improving your physical, emotional and spiritual health. We've gone through the home and health benefits of essential oils. Aromatherapy is simply the application of these oils to improve your health, mostly as a supplement to existing medical treatment.

Plants possess multiple beneficial compounds and chemicals to protect themselves from insects and viruses. The most dominant ingredients from the oils are extracted from medicinal plants or herbs through the process of distillation. It is subsequently combined with alcohol to retain its qualities and strength. The end result is a thoroughly concentrated formula that can easily be combined with various neutral substances (known as carriers) such as almond oil or coconut oil, before massaging into the skin.

History of Aromatherapy

Though the spotlight fell on it quite late, aromatherapy has been practiced for more than 5,000 years across multiple global cultures. Natural healers and those preferring natural treatments are invariably drawn to aromatherapy on account of its all-natural, no side effects goodness. Many essential oils are known for their antimicrobial and anti-inflammatory characteristics. Its main uses include pain management, enjoying a more relaxed and peaceful sleep, eliminating stress, combating symptoms of stress and depression, soothing tense muscles and joints and even fighting cancer.

There are more than 40 various grades of essential aromatherapy oils in the market today that are widely used in home, beauty and wellness products. The uses of essentials oils have evolved through the ages according to the evolution of mankind and culture. Once used for spiritual and cultural rituals, its use spread to health and wellness, beauty products, and today, household purposes. What was once seen as a magic potion by ancient Egyptians, today magically cleans our homes and beautifies us. Though the uses have changed and evolved over the years, the intrinsic goodness of essential oils is intact.

Like most wellness and beauty essentials, it is challenging to determine the earliest origins of aromatherapy. Essential oils have been utilized for ages by ancient Chinese, Greeks, Jews, Romans and Egyptians as fragrances, beauty and wellness products. Certain cultures and civilizations also used these oils for spiritual purposes and specific rituals. They were an integral part of the spiritual rituals of several cultures including Egyptian and Jew cultures.

The ancient Egyptians used cedarwood, myrrh, clove and other natural oils for embalming the dead. The opening of a tomb in the20th century lead to several startling discoveries related to the use of essential oils in ancient Egyptian culture. Several traces of essential oils were found on flawlessly intact body parts. The fragrance, though not very overpowering, could still be experienced. While some oils were crudely distilled by erstwhile Egyptians, others were used in an infused form.

The Egyptians also took to essential oils for creating herbal and medicinal portions for spiritual, health and cosmetic utilization. Essential oils were also a huge source of fragrance for the ancient Egyptian community.

Want some fun trivia? Ancient Egyptian men placed a cone of solid fragrance on their head. The solid cone would slowly start melting into a liquid form and completely envelop their body. Ingenious? You bet!

Not to be outdone by the Egyptians, the Greeks too took to essential oils in a big way. Perfumes play a huge role in Greek mythology since they also were aware of the medicinal properties of plants. Hippocrates, referred to as the "father of medicine" undertook fumigations of oils for healing as well as fragrance.

It is interesting to note that an ancient Greek perfumer known as Megallus made a fragrance termed as "megaleion," which included a fat based oil and myrrh. It was used for several purposes, including for its all-powerful aroma, healing powers and anti-inflammatory properties.

Later, the Roman Empire emulated the practices of the Egyptians and Greeks. It led Dioscorides to author an entire book known as De Materia Medica, which described, among other things, the characteristics of about 500 known plant species. The process of distillation was also briefly studied by Dioscorides.

In the 14th century, the fatal Black Death hit hard, and millions succumbed to it. Herbal and natural medicinal preparations were heavily sought to battle the disastrous disease. Some people successfully avoided the plague owing to their close contact with the essential oils.

During the 15th century, the process of distillation gained momentum, and several plants were utilized for creating essential oils through distillation, including rose, rosemary, frankincense and sage. The growth in printing and publication led to the growth of books related to plants and herbs, which led to even more interest and awareness about aromatherapy.

By mid-16th century, people started buying oils at what was known as the apothecary. This is when plenty of today's essential oils first became known to people. Perfumery became an artistic discipline. The art form thrived by mid-19thcentury when people realized the potency of fragrances. Women got their jewelers to create exclusive, ornamental bottles for storing their favorite fragrances.

A noted alchemist, thinker and doctor, Paracelsus first used the term "essence," and later shifted his focus from alchemy to using plants for medicinal purposes.

In the 20th century, the process of segregating essential oil constituents became widely used for the creation of artificial drugs, medicines and chemicals. It was concluded that separating these constituents and individually making use of them in a synthetic form would not just be more economical but also possesses plenty of therapeutic benefits.

The 21st century has seen a sudden demand for more organic, natural and earthy products. The back to basics philosophy has people looking for more natural and plant-based products for their health, wellness and beauty. Essential oils have therefore captured the interest of the new-age community looking for natural oil based therapies, cosmetics and fragrances.

Though the popularity and widespread use of essentials oils didn't stop, the industrial revolution reduced its application in daily life. The advent of the internet, coupled with the publication of books related to the subject and other periodicals has stimulated interest in aromatherapy and essential oils for all purposes.

Rene-Maurice Gattefosse, a French chemist, first used lavender oil for treating a hand burn. He later extensively studied the medicinal benefits of lavender oil in treating all kinds of skin troubles, including wounds and infections. Gattefosse is known as the father of aromatherapy for his contribution to the field of using essential oils as alternate and natural medicines.

Other eminent 20th-century aromatherapy experts were Jean Valnet and Robert B. Tisserand. Austrian biochemist Madam Marguerite Maury is credited with being an avid practitioner of aromatherapy for the purpose of making cosmetics. Robert B. Tisserand's book, *The Art of Aromatherapy*, was the first published English book dedicated to aromatherapy.

Though Gattfosse's primary intention was to treat the wounded soldiers of World War I, the uses of these essential oils began to spread rapidly. It became hugely popular with holistic medicine practitioners, who were looking for more natural treatments than chemical laden medicines. Beauticians, masseurs and therapists from all over Europe began to extensively use essential oils in their treatments.

Aromatherapy didn't gain popularity until late 19th century when essential oils slowly started trickling their way into everyday use in the form of candles, beauty lotions and other scented products. There are several trained professionals such as therapists, nutritionists, naturopaths, massage therapists and aromatherapists who specifically deal with the various benefits of essential oils.

Essential oils have also been used to reduce anxiety, stress and tension during childbirth. Another study discovered that women who utilized aromatherapy during labor and childbirth experienced far less pain on the whole.

How Does Aromatherapy Work?

When you inhale essential oils through the nose, the aroma molecules are gradually transported through the nasal cavity lining by olfactory glands (housed in the inner nose) to the limbic system located in the brain. This limbic system is directly responsible for impacting our autonomic nervous system and also the vital endocrine system.

The body's endocrine system is a primary force for the functioning of our body. It comprises hormone-secreting glands that release the hormones into our bloodstream. When they are passed into the body's bloodstream, these hormones act as chemical mediators and balance several bodily functions including metabolism, emotional health, mood and development.

The autonomic nervous system operates involuntarily, mostly without our awareness of control. It links the brain and spine to other organs by electric impulses, which regulate primary physical reactions such as sweating, salivating, increase in heartbeat and sexual stimulation. Inhalation is known to be one of the fastest and easiest ways to deliver healing elements of oils into our body.

They travel through the nasal cavity and gain direct access to our brain, through which they work their benefits on other systems that directly control the body. This pretty conclusively explains why we link certain smells with very specific emotions. Ever noticed how a peculiar smell triggers a memory or induces specific emotions, while you remain baffled about why that happens? This is how inhaling beneficial essential oils impacts our body's vital systems, and influences its overall functionality. Thus, essential oils can have an intense impact on our physical and psychological state.

When rubbed into the skin, essential oils are absorbed into the body's bloodstream. From the bloodstream, they are transported to different parts of the body or organs, where they begin working their magic. Some essential oils are known to permeate the bloodstream-brain barrier and directly enter our limbic system, where again they impact our autonomic nervous and endocrine systems.

There are several factors that influence the absorption capacity of essential oils into the skin, such as gently massage the area before applying essential oil to it. This will boost circulation within that region, and facilitate better absorption of the oil. Another factor that facilitates better absorption and circulation is heat.

Irrespective of whether they are used topically or inhaled, essential oils can bring about a transformation in our physical, emotional, spiritual and mental condition by stimulating the body's natural responses. For instance, most essential oil blends are created with a mix of topical and inhalation use in mind, which increases the efficacy.

What are the Primary Uses of Aromatherapy?

Aromatherapy is a holistic health and wellness therapy that is used for facilitating relaxation and soothing stress and anxiety. It is also known to combat a wide range of physical and psychological conditions such as wounds and burns, depression, sleep disorders and infections.

Extensive research in the field of aromatherapy has revealed that aromatherapy oils are packed with plenty of natural sedatives and stimulating agents, plus elements that help boost our immune system and effectively control the nervous system (PDQ Integrative, Alternative, and Complementary Therapies Editorial Board 2005). It has been concluded that there is a correlation between the usage of aromatherapy oils and a feel-good effect on the body's limbic system. It helps us better manage our moods, behaviors and emotional responses.

One of the most important points to keep in mind before using aromatherapy is to stick only with using pure, high quality, top grade oils that do not feature artificial ingredients or scents. The results of aromatherapy are almost always based on the grade of the oil you use and the quantity in which it is used.

Here are a few common uses of aromatherapy

-Persistent stress, tension, nervousness and anxiety

- Chronic depression

- Muscle soreness or pain

- Respiratory ailments

- Digestive system disorders

- Menstrual cramps/menopause symptoms

- Skin disorders, including skin rashes, acne, bites, wounds and cellulite

- Blood sugar regulation

- Malaise and fatigue

Is Aromatherapy a Safe Practice?

Aromatherapy is not a licensed practice in the United States, which means that though other health professionals (licensed) may practice aromatherapy as an alternate form of healing and wellness, it isn't a specially designated discipline yet. Generally, massage therapists, counselors and other healthcare professionals are trained in the practice of aromatherapy. Before practicing aromatherapy in any form for treating a disorder or illness, it is best to consult with your physician or a licensed medical practitioner.

Also, if you've started using aromatherapy as an alternative or supplementary healing practice, keep your doctor in the loop about it. Do not simply stop the conventional medical treatment, and start aromatherapy without consulting a medical practitioner, and depending exclusively on aromatherapy to help you gain glowing health.

People with the following conditions should not use aromatherapy until they consult with a certified and experienced medical practitioner.

- People suffering from chronic ailments such as asthma, respiration-related allergies, chronic lung ailments and other similar lung or respiration-related disorders. Essential oils may trigger breathing pathway spasms.

- People suffering from skin allergies should refrain from using essential oils without proper consultation since it can lead to skin irritation.

- Pregnant women should use caution before using aromatherapy since some essential oils such as rosemary lead to contractions of the uterus. Consult a midwife or doula before usage.

The expert and insightful advice offered by these professionals may help you determine if aromatherapy is worth practicing and can help enhance your health. Also, ensure that the oils aren't orally ingested in any form. Many of these oils can be lethal if consumed orally, though a few can be ingested.

Bear in mind that kids below the age of 7 should avoid using aromatherapy owing to the highly sensitive characteristics of the oil. Exercise caution while using oil near sensitive regions such as the eyes, nose, mouth, etc. It can lead to skin irritation and other unpleasant effects.

Aromatherapy in Daily Life

1. Brighten the mood a bit —Add lavender, rose and orange essential oils into a diffuser to lighten up the stress in a room, and make the atmosphere more tranquil, serene and positive. Keep some lavender or orange oil ready when you get back from work. Just use a diffuser or light a candle to create a nice, soothing and de-stressing ambiance.

2. Stay alert while driving – Stay alert while driving by inhaling a combination of any of these essential oils – lavender, frankincense, lemongrass and lemon or peppermint. The aroma emitting from the essential oils helps keep the senses active and prevents you from feeling lethargic or sleepy. Well, how about adding a few drops of these oils to the car freshener to keep you up and alert while driving?

3. Create a nice, relaxing room – Want to create a relaxing ambiance in your break or nap room? Use chamomile, cedarwood or lavender oil for a stress-less, relaxing, positive and soothing space where you can head to for recharging your energy. The aroma will trigger your positive and feel-good hormones, which will help you feel less stressed and more relaxed.

4. Preserve fruit freshness – Preserve the goodness of fruits by washing them and retain their freshness with the help of grapefruit oil. Wash the fruits thoroughly in water, and later store them by adding a few drops of grapefruit oil to it to retain its freshness and goodness.

What Are the Different Methods of Inhaling Essential Oils?

Spray – Spraying a few drops of essential oil mixed with water is one of the best ways to use it. Simply add a few drops of essential oil into any water solution. Shake it properly, and subsequently spray it into the air for fresher, purer and cleaner smelling air. It will lend a pleasant mood and ambiance to the space.

For instance, to create a festival cheer, you can spray a few drops of pine oil into the air. Similarly, spraying peppermint essential oil triggers alertness and concentration. Shake the container well before use to spray an effective proportion of water and essential oil.

Steam – Add a few drops of essential oil to a large bowl of boiling water, and convert it into vaporizing oil immediately. Cover your head and face completely with a towel and breathe the oil and water mixture kept just below you. Close your eyes to avoid any damage to the internal vision membranes or prevent irritation. Use a few drops of eucalyptus essential oil in warm water as a natural remedy against sinus and other respiratory infections.

Note that this method isn't recommended for children below 8 years of age. When older children are using this method of essential oil inhalation, they can use their swimming goggles for protection.

Dry Evaporation – Multiple drops of essential oil can be added to a cotton ball and left to enter the air. If it's more intense doses you are seeking, simply sniff the cotton ball or place it near you for continuous exposure.

Diffuser – Essential oils are kept in this handy device, at times combined with water or heat (to facilitate evaporation).

How Do I Prepare an Aromatherapy Solution?

As a general principle, essential oils should always be diluted with a carrier, which can either be water or neutral oil such as vegetable oil in a concentration percentage of not more than 3-6%. For instance, if you are using a single teaspoon of carrier, you should add not more than 2-3 drops of essential oil.

For applying on the body or for massage, a 1 percent solution of essential oil is a good concentration. Do not go beyond 1% percent for massages as it may not be very safe in a high concentration. If you are utilizing water as a carrier base, do not forget to shake the solution effectively before using.

What are the Necessary Precautions While Using Essential Oils for Aromatherapy?

Essential oils are packed with natural goodness and have multiple virtues. However, there is some caution to be exercised while using them. First, do not use them in an undiluted form, especially near the mucous membranes or sensitive areas like the eyes.

Second, they aren't to be ingested generally speaking. However, consult a qualified practitioner as some types of essential oils can be safely ingested in small quantities. As a thumb rule, never orally consume it until you consult with an experienced and qualified practitioner.

Keep essential oils out of reach of children. Also, if you're applying any of these essential oils to the skin for the first time, conduct a patch test in a small area to check the skin's sensitivity to the oil. Go ahead and apply it on the skin only if a particular patch of your skin responds well to the oil. Essential oils are powerful solutions and may cause skin problems if you have highly sensitive skin.

Never use essential oils on their own when applying to the skin. Always mix it with a suitable carrier oil before applying.

Why is Aromatherapy Massage Considered to be Beneficial?

Massage is considered to be one of the best ways of enjoying the benefits of aromatherapy because it not just helps you gain the therapeutic benefits of the essential oil but also gives you the goodness of massage. When combined with the therapeutic powers of essential oils, massage can offer even more revitalizing powers for energizing multiple organs, including the muscles, glands and skin.

Massage boosts blood circulation and flow of lymph while helping the body get rid of harmful toxins. Since essential oils are proven emotion influencers, aromatherapy massage offers a complete body and mind treatment. It is known to fight depression, and offer an overall positive mind state.

Massage with essential oils is especially effective in treating women's health issues, such as PMS and menopause disorders. It can also help alleviate the more mild forms of anxiety and depression, insomnia, emotional imbalances, headaches, muscle aches, etc. Most essential oils perfectly nourish the skin. They balance the secretion of sebum and improve the tones of the skin by acting on the function of the capillaries. Also, plant essences can be used in hair and head preparations because they prevent the occurrence of dandruff and stimulate hair growth.

If you apply them without massage, essential oils help to eliminate fungus, itching, or herpes sores. If you use them for steam inhalations, you can alleviate the cold and flu, as well as a cough and inflammation of the tonsils or throat.

In addition to the fact that essential oils are healing, only by smelling them do we mend our mood and feel better. This is because the sense of smell is associated with the limbic system - an area in the brain that deals with emotions and memory. And that's exactly the explanation of the mysterious possibilities of aromatherapy and psychotherapy that helps with emotional and mental imbalances.

Essential oils such as marjoram, sandalwood, lavender and frankincense trigger a neurotransmitter known as serotonin that helps the body feel relaxed and sleepy naturally. This is exactly why essential oils or aromatherapy massage is so popular when it comes to natural remedies for stress, anxiety, tension, nervousness, psychological disorders and insomnia. It effectively reduces plenty of symptoms and conditions related to these orders in the long-term.

10 Power Packed Health Benefits of Aroma Therapy

Boosts Memory

One of the most common conditions related to the memory is memory loss or Alzheimer's. Aromatherapy is widely used as an alternative therapy for Alzheimer's since it impedes the condition from worsening. That being said, it is also great for boosting the memory, concentration and focus for students. Aromatherapy is often used for memory boosting purposes among youngsters. It helps enhance the memory capacity of a person for a specific time after the therapy.

Sage oil is considered to be the best when it comes to stimulating boosting memory powers with aromatherapy.

Decreases Headaches

Don't we all suffer from headaches periodically? The horrible ones can totally stop us from functioning normally. Rather than relying on chemical laden pharmaceuticals or buying expensive massage treatments, use a natural solution that's available in your home. You will not just experience relief from your headache, but also gain freedom from anxiety, nervousness, stress and insomnia. That's a lot of birds with one stone! The most effective aromatherapy oils for battling headaches, anxiety and sleep disorders are peppermint, sandalwood, rosemary and eucalyptus. For best results, mix any of these oils with carrier oil (coconut, almond or sesame oil), and massage it gently on the scalp, forehead or temples.

Headaches and stress can also be the cause of insomnia and disturbed sleeping patterns. Fortunately, aromatherapy comes to the rescue again. The use of specific essential oils can help you regulate your sleep patterns, effectively align your circadian rhythms, sleep soundly through the night, and leave you feeling bright and invigorated the next day.

Some of the most effective essential oils when it comes to regulating your sleep patterns are sandalwood, lavender, rose, ylang-ylang, chamomile, benzoin and marjoram. These oils are known to be excellent natural sedatives that induce a feeling of relaxation and drowsiness when you use them just before going to bed. You can either light an aroma candle, diffuse them in the air, have them massaged on your back or have a few drops sprayed on the pillow. They work like natural, magical sleep potions.

Facilitates Digestion

Aromatherapy can be used to treat a range of digestive conditions including bloating and constipation. It helps facilitate faster metabolism so your food can digest faster. Which is the best essential oil for aromatherapy related to digestive issues? Ginger, orange, lemon, clary sage and fennel. Many ailments we suffer are directly or indirectly related to the functioning of our digestive system, which is why it is important to keep it functioning effectively.

In addition to facilitating digestion, essential oils such as cinnamon, lemon, eucalyptus, frankincense and more help improve the body's overall immune system. Thus, they should be a staple in your home if you are looking for boosted immunity and glowing health.

Boosting Energy Levels

Feeling drained and low on energy? It is time to recharge your batteries with aromatherapy. We all need that extra energy and enthusiasm to go with our daily chores. Can you imagine what the harmful substances such as caffeine, cigarettes and the so-called energy boosting pills do to your body? A balanced diet, sufficient physical activity and aromatherapy is a great combination for keeping your energy levels constantly high. Stimulate your physical and mental faculties without resorting to harmful substances.

The most beneficial essential oils when it comes to awarding yourself a much-needed energy boost is cinnamon, tea tree, cardamom, jasmine, black pepper and rosemary. Including these essential oils in your daily life will keep you feeling energized, positive and rejuvenated throughout the day.

Facilitates Healing

Many essential oils act as stimulants for boosting your body's healing capacity, due inducing higher quantities of oxygen and proper blood circulation. More oxygen and a vigorous blood flow ensure a faster healing process. This is especially true for postoperative patients or those who have had surgeries performed on them. Aromatherapy is also good for people who've just come out of an illness.

Many essential oils possess anti-microbial properties that safeguard the body and expedite its healing process. The most popular essential oils used for aromatherapy when it comes to healing goals are lavender, rosehip and calendula. These oils are also beneficial when it comes to healing the skin in disorders such as eczema.

Chapter Four: 18 Essential Oils That Are a Must in Your Home Lab

Does essential oil automatically conjure up images of pricey and exotic oils that are to be used only by the rich and famous? You couldn't be any more wrong. Here is a list of 10 handy, effective, easily available and affordable essential oils that are popular for their multiple applications and potency. These oils have made their way into the list on account of being packed with goodness and a number of health advantages. They are not just laden with superficial aromatic properties, but also offer tons of other benefits while helping you feel good from within. Here are the 18 must-have essential oils for your home lab.

1. Cinnamon Oil

One of the most popular essential oils that is known for its versatility and multi-purpose applications, cinnamon oil has a nice, sweet, warm and spicy fragrance that lends a seductive and exotic aroma. It's a staple in many Asian spice drawers, and the smell is at best cozily homey and familiar.

Did you know that cinnamon oil is one amongst the world's oldest essential oils? Its use dates back to 1550 BC as chronicled in the ancient Egyptian Ebers Papyrus, an eminent medical text of its time. The oil is extracted from the leaf as well as the bark of *Cinnamomum verum*.

Cinnamon was a hugely hot item during the erstwhile era. Its supply was majorly controlled by Arab merchants, as a result of which they kept their supply source (Sri Lanka and India) a top secret. It was the prerogative of a select few, owing to the high price and luxurious uses. It was most sought after by the royals and western elites.

Luckily, we do not have to worry about the price today. Today, cinnamon oil is a must-have in your home lab. It can be used for various purposes, including clearing up the chest in case of cold. Cinnamon essential oil is also known to be effective for offering relief from sore muscles and aches, courtesy its analgesic characteristics. It is also a potent antiseptic, while also acting as a powerful preservative (all packed with natural goodness). The aroma is so alluring and overpowering that you'll almost feel like eating this nice smelling oil.

Other health benefits of cinnamon oil include its anti-inflammatory properties. It is also a widely used antioxidant that is known to fight the body's toxins. Its potential goes as far as being effective for battling heart disorders and neurological ailments. And that's just the tip of the iceberg of this immensely beneficial essential oil. Who can resist the sweet, pleasant, and positive fragrance of these oils?

2. Lavender Oil

Lavender oil has so many benefits that it's almost synonymous with essential oils or aromatherapy. It is virtually impossible to ignore the goodness of lavender essential oil. So, let's get it straight, the lavender essential oil that is utilized in our daily life comes only from a single type of lavender from about 40 odd lavender species. While all species vary in characteristics (each contains varying proportions of camphor, eucalyptol, and other components), on average it's packed with several highly beneficial and quality components, which makes it an essential oil staple.

The *Lavandula angustifolia* plant has a fragrance that's a pleasant mix of fresh, spring floral, soothing and clean. These are the properties that have made the plant a staple for perfumes, soaps, beauty products and air fresheners. If you're just getting started with aromatherapy and do not want something too overpowering, lavender is a lovely beginner essential oil. It isn't simply preferred owing to its signature, classic scent but also because of its sheer versatility. Lavender essential oil can be used in everything from beauty care products to relaxing spa-style pampering treatments to cleaners.

What are the benefits of lavender, you ask? It is a natural sedative and a highly beneficial anti-anxiety fighter. Lavender essential oil is packed with anti-bacterial and anti-inflammatory properties, while also being a known immune system booster and antispasmodic. It is especially useful for people having trouble with getting good sleep or those suffering from stress or anxiety.

This versatile and affordable essential oil has a million different uses in your daily life, including that of a natural and wholesome beauty product. Mix about five to six drops of lavender essential oil in a spoonful of carrier oil. Apply it on your skin for great results! You can experiment on a patch of skin, and according to the results increase the concentration or proportion of lavender oil vis-à-vis carrier oil. It has already discussed ways in which lavender oil can be used for various home, health and beauty purposes in the above chapters.

There are so many ways to include lavender essential oil in your daily routine.

Add a few drops of lavender essential oil to shampoos, conditioners, lotions and other beauty and skincare products for a wow fragrance.

Want to make your own pampering, home spa treatment? Mix a cup of Epsom salt with 4-5 drops of lavender oil and add to your hot bath. You'llbe forgiven for feeling like Cleopatra.

Fancy a homemade, all-natural body scrub? Add a few drops of lavender essential oil to sugar/salt and coconut.

Lavender essential oil can be used for a relaxing and soothing back massage. You can also use it as part of a daily pampering routine. Simply rub a few drops of lavender oil on the feet soles before retreating to bed or spray a few drops of it mixed with water on your pillow. Make a DIY room freshener by diffusing lavender into the air to fight stale odors.

3. Lemongrass Oil

Well, lemongrass has more uses than lending your Thai curry a distinct flavor. It's one of the most popular tropical East Asian grass plants from South India and Sri Lanka, which needs a nice, warm climate to flourish. The best part about lemongrass is all its parts are useful. Almost every component of the plant is beneficial either for making tea or cleaning products or treating ailments such as fever or wound healing.

Apart from featuring a positive, energetic and feel-good scent, lemongrass has myriad medicinal benefits. It has a nice mild, herbal lemon aroma that's hard to miss. It is also believed to potentially impede the growth of cancerous cells in the body.

Research has pointed out that lemongrass oil possesses ant-bacterial and anti-inflammatory properties (Naik, et al. 2010). It acts as a powerful insect repellent as well as fights stubborn dandruff yeast with effectiveness. If nothing, add a few drops of lemongrass essential oil to your bath and witness the change in your mood!

Looking for an inexpensive aroma-sauna therapy? Add a couple of drops of lemongrass, lavender or any other preferred essential oil fragrance into about two water cups inside the sauna for a wonderfully relaxing and cheap sauna therapy. You do not have to spend a fortune to feel like royalty if you have access to a few essential oils and a tiny bit of creativity.

4. Tea Tree Oil

Tea tree oil is enjoying the attention that's coming its way from the world of beauty and cosmetics right now, with good reason. It's naturally good and beneficial, and not just another hyped, overpriced cosmetic product. Tea tree grows mainly in Australia, and native Australians were known to use it for curing common cold, coughs, wounds and skin ailments. It is also known to possess anticancer properties.

Tea tree oil is also believed to be effective against dandruff, oral bacteria and combating the influenza virus. It is an excellent natural agent against acne and other skin ailments, owing to its moisturizing abilities. Try adding a few drops of tea tree oil to a drugstore mouthwash for pleasant smelling, fresh breath.

Some little-known uses of tea tree essential oil include:

Add a couple of drops near the base of your ear for treating ear pain or infections in a natural manner.

Suffering from skin rashes or itching? Dab a drop of tea tree oil on your skin as a natural remedy for itching. Include some drops (2-3) of tea tree essential oil into home created natural shampoos and rises.

You can also mix about 5 drops of tea tree oil into a homemade cleaning spray for getting rid of germs and harmful bacteria. Also, apply about 3-4 drops of tea tree oil diluted in a tablespoon of coconut oil on your feet once or twice a day for preventing athlete's foot.

5. Peppermint Oil

Peppermint already boasts of widespread benefits in our home and health. It is almost everywhere, from your mouthwash to shampoo to toothpaste and chewing gum. However, few of us know the actual benefits and goodness of peppermint that makes it a staple in these products.

Peppermint is a powerful antispasmodic, antioxidant, antiviral and antimicrobial natural compound that is comprised predominantly of menthone and menthol. The essential oil is believed to offer amazing results in cases of stress, tension, anxiety and headaches. Peppermint essential oil also pacifies nausea, boosts memory and concentration and combats skin pain.

Use it in any lip care product, and you'll be treated to incredibly healthy and refreshed looking lips.

Here are some other uses of peppermint essential oil

Apply a drop of peppermint oil to your forehead to eliminate headaches. Avoid letting it into your eyes though.

Mix 5-6 drops of water to a 16oz. water spray and utilize it as a natural cooling agent when temperatures rise. You can also take a whiff of the pleasant, cooling fragrance to eliminate nausea.

A couple of drops of peppermint essential oil added to your feet soles can help fight fever.

Add 6-7 drops of peppermint oil in a 16-oz. spray bottle to spray in the molding region for keeping pests at bay.

Want an amazingly easy to make yet super effective natural balm? Combine peppermint oil and lavender oil. Here's the method of preparation.

Ingredients

5-6 drops each of lavender essential oil and peppermint essential oil

1/2 c coconut oil

2 T marshmallow Root

3 T beeswax

2 T calendula

Method of preparation

Heat oven to 200 degrees Celsius (approximately 390 degrees Fahrenheit) and switch off. Melt all coconut oil on very low heat and mix with herbs. Let it set on low heat for about five minutes. Transfer the mixture into the oven. Allow the herbs to assimilate into the mixture for more than four hours. Remove all herbs from the oil. Now, place the oil on a pan and treat it to low heat.

Include the wax and allow it to melt on low heat. Add the lavender and peppermint essential oils. Add a few more drops of the oils if you want a stronger fragrance. Pour the entire mixture into a clean storage container.

Want to be treated to instant café style mint cocoa? Well, just add 2 drops of peppermint essential oil into warm cocoa for a nice, inexpensive choco-mint drink to keep you warm during biting cold winters.

6. Eucalyptus Oil

Ever experienced a jammed nose? Eucalyptus oil is extremely useful for clearing blocked nasal passages. It has a very overpowering and pungent smell (much like a balm ointment or Vicks). The smell is minty and pretty much like camphor, which is why it is particularly effective against cold. Apply a few drops of eucalyptus oil on a handkerchief for relief from common cold.

Alternately, you can add a few drops to a cotton ball or thin cloth and place it near you while sleeping to get relief from a persistent cough and cold. Eucalyptus is also an effective pesticide that is known to act effectively against mites, fungus, and weeds. It is also beneficial prevention against malaria-causing parasites. If you want your space to feel cleaner, fresher and more purified, diffuse a few drops of eucalyptus oil within the room.

In addition to being an effective natural remedy for cough and cold and a known space freshener and cleanser, eucalyptus oil is also used as a pantry moth repellent. Leave a few drops of it in closed spaces that are prone to be attacked by bugs, and witness how it works effectively to keep the pests at bay.

Since Eucalyptus is packed with antimicrobial and antibacterial properties, it makes for an excellent natural cleanser. It can also be used as a natural expectorant for fighting respiratory congestion.

Here are some ways to use eucalyptus oil in everyday life.

Mix 10 drops of eucalyptus oil with 2 tablespoons of liquid soap and warm water. Use this mixture for mopping your floor and making it look sparkling clean.

Mix about 3-4 drops of eucalyptus oil with a tablespoon of warm coconut oil and gently rub it on the chest for instant relief against cough and cold.

Add a few drops (about 5-6) of eucalyptus essential oil to the diffuser for treating your home to fresher and cleaner air.

Combine 5 drops of eucalyptus oil along with 5 drops of tea tree oil in a 16 oz. spray bottle of water. Spray it on the shower to impede mold growth in the shower and other parts of your home. You can also mix a few drops (3-4) of eucalyptus essential oil in a pet shampoo for keeping fleas at bay.

7. Clary Sage Oil

Clary sage oil possesses multiple benefits and characteristics that helps the skin. It is a popular antiseptic and antibacterial element that is known to facilitate circulation throughout the body. Since it has a nice, non-overwhelming fragrance, clary sage is great when combined with more overpowering skin care ingredients.

The plant has been hailed since long ago for its ability to regulate hormones and working as an effective natural anti-depressant. In a 2014 study, it was concluded that clary sage helped in reducing the body's cortisol levels and enhanced the thyroid hormonal levels (Lee, Cho and Kang 2014). When combined with lavender, clary sage can be effective for massages, while also reducing menstrual cramps and persistent pain.

Clary sage's first recorded use dates back to the Egyptians, though it didn't attain popularity until the medieval era. Its oil is extracted through a process of distillation (flower tops and leaves). In the medieval age, it acted as an effective remedy for people looking to treat issues related to vision, while also being a popular wine flavor.

8. Rosemary Oil

Rosemary oil is similar to the flavor that's used to enhance Italian treats. What many do not know is that rosemary essential oil is brilliant for skin care and acts as a fabulous natural preservative.

Inhaling rosemary oil can help with blood pressure, breathing rate and heart rate. It is also a known immune system booster, apart from enhancing human brain waves. Rosemary facilitates the component of a nervous system that manages organ functionality, thus ensuring that all vital organs function effectively. Rosemary oil is also an effective stress reducer. You just need to diffuse a few drops of the essential oil in the air for it to work its charm. Want you home to smell like a flourishing, green jungle? Well, simply combine eucalyptus and rosemary oil and spread it all over the space.

9. Sweet Orange Oil

The fact that its sweet, fruity, pleasant aroma is loved by many only accentuates the goodness of this sweet-smelling, multi-purpose essential oil. A single whiff of this energizing oil can make you feel instantly upbeat, positive and energetic. Research confirms that sweet orange essential oil is great when it comes to reducing stress and anxiety. It is known to reduce heavy breathing and rapid pulse rates while helping you feel good.

Here are some ways in which you can add this sweet-smelling oil into your everyday life.

Add a drops of sweet orange oil to a tablespoon of coconut oil and gently massage your tummy for a quick and effective relief against a stomach upset. You can make a stronger mix if you want a more powerful fragrance and effect.

Mix 2-3 drops of sweet orange essential oil and a tablespoon of coconut oil. Rub it on the chest to get rid of cold. Diffuse 3 drops of wild orange and lavender oil each for a relaxing effect and super amazing smell.

Diffuse around 5-6 drops of orange essential oil to cleanse the air of microbes, bacterial and other harmful elements.

Combine 3 drops each of sweet orange and peppermint essential oil with about 20 drops of carrier oil. Gently massage this mixture on the back to boost concentration and focus. It can be used on older children to help them in their academics and other learning, memory or knowledge related activities.

10. Lemon Oil

Lemon essence is utilized in everything from household cleaners to flavored water to hand soaps. The fragrance is known to be fresh, fruity, zesty, clean and non-overpowering. Notwithstanding the fact that many products all over the world use artificial lemon flavors in their products, there's still a huge following for original lemon flavors. It's not just a superb anti-oxidant but is also a worldwide symbol of freshness and sparkling cleanliness.

Packed with goodness, lemon essential oil is known to possess potent antibacterial properties and acts as an effective antiseptic. Dilute a few drops of lemon oil to create a powerful skin care product. It effectively battles wrinkles and skin tone and promotes blood circulation to get a natural and flawless looking skin. Lemon essential oil is also popular for its anti-inflammatory and skin replenishing properties.

Want a quick, effective and inexpensive mood booster? Chuck those pizzas and cupcakes, lemon oil is the solution. Lemon oil is an effective antidepressant. One whiff of lemon essential oil is enough to make you feel all positive and energetic.

Looking for some ideas to include lemon essential oil into your everyday life?

Add a drop of lemon essential oil and a drop of honey to get instant relief from cough and sore throat.

Diffuse 4-5 drops of lemon essential oil within the room for eliminating foul odors and boost your mood.

For getting rid of stubbornly sticky residue from surfaces, use 2-3 drops of lemon essential oil. This remedy can also be useful for removing gum from a cloth or even hair.

Combine 4 drops with 4 oz. of liquid dish wash for eliminating that extra stubborn grease from utensils.

If you aren't a big fan of chemical and alcohol-laden hand sanitizers, you can make a nice, natural, citrus based hand sanitizer using lemon essential oil. Here's how.

Ingredients

14 drops of sweet orange essential oil

14 drops of lemon essential oil

14 drops of lime essential oil

9 drops of tea tree essential oil

½ teaspoon of Vitamin E oil

1 tablespoon witch hazel

Spray bottles

½ cup aloe vera gel (pure)

Add all essential oils and the natural preservative (Vitamin E) to a measuring cup, and shake everything thoroughly. Include witch hazel to the mixture gently and mix again. Now gently add aloe vera and mix. Store in travel bottles or a spray. On first use, the sanitizer may feel highly sticky, but the solution will soak really quickly without leaving behind a sticky residue. The natural hand sanitizer will not just smell good but keeps your hands nice and soft. This natural, citrus-based hand sanitizer is also safe for children above the age of 3.

11. Sandalwood Oil

Sandalwood essential oil is another staple, must-have in your essential oils box for its sheer versatility and benefits. It is effective against emotional issues and is also a great spiritual ambiance enhancer. Need more reasons to stock up on sandalwood oil? It is great for skin and is widely used for making natural, alcohol-free perfumes.

Since ancient times, sandalwood has been the essential oil of choice for spiritual purposes. It is known to be intensely grounding and is beneficial for activating chakra points.

Sandalwood helps maintain a sense of emotional balance and inner peace by calming the senses. It is good for fighting stress-related and psychological conditions such as depression, anxiety, low self-confidence and nervousness. Sandalwood essential oil is also a known sexual stimulator.

Aromatically, the oil is intense, sweet yet somewhat woody. Its fragrance is universally popular, which is why it is widely used in perfumes, beauty products and toiletries. It is also an excellent base fragrance that evens out other blends.

12. Myrrh Oil

Myrrh essential oil has been utilized since ancient times for its wonderful cosmetic, fragrance and medicinal properties. In Christian mythology, it is recognized to be one of the gifts given to Jesus by the wise kings. Therefore, even today myrrh is closely associated with spirituality and is used as incense for spiritual fragrance purposes. It is also known to be an excellent oral health agent. It can be used to create natural, home-made mouth rinses and oral care products. Before adding it to any oral product, ensure that you consult an experienced aromatherapy or essential oil practitioner.

On its own, the aroma of myrrh can be pleasant yet overpowering. You can use another milder essential oil such as frankincense to neutralize the powerful fragrance of myrrh. The fragrance of myrrh can be best described as woody and balsamic, which makes it an excellent base aroma note for mixing with other notes in creating a spiritual atmosphere or perfuming a space for festivals.

13. Frankincense Oil

Frankincense essential oil has been utilized since ancient times for its exceptional medicinal, fragrance and skin care properties. It has multiple spiritual purposes (since it is referred to as one of the gifts offered by the wise men to baby Jesus), dating back to applications during the erstwhile era.

It is most often used for making perfumes, incense, and to supplying fragrance or cleansing rooms. Frankincense is also known to be an effective expectorant and often used to gain relief against respiratory disorders and cough. The nature of its aroma can be described as fresh, pure and sweet, while also being earthy, warm and spicy.

You can make natural incense, room fresheners and all kinds of spiritual blends with Frankincense Essential Oil.

On a psychological level, the fragrance can be extremely calming, soothing, relaxing and uplifting. The note makes you feel good on an emotional plane, without causing a sedating effect.

14. Basil Oil

If you're looking for an essential oil that makes you feel instantly stimulated, alert and focused, basil it is! Basil is intensely energizing, and that's just the beginning of its goodness. It is also an effective remedy for cold and cough for its amazing anti-viral properties. Looking for a natural cure for headaches?Basil, it is again. Since basil oil contains linalool, it also acts as an effective insect repellent. If you find the essence or fragrance of basil too overpowering, use it as a blend.

15. Roman Chamomile Oil

Roman chamomile essential oil is highly effective for combating issues related to loneliness, anxiety, depression, post trauma shock and nervousness. It helps restore a sense of calmness and emotional balance. It is also a workable, natural solution for eliminating anger, impulsiveness and irritability.

It is believed to be one of the safest essential oils for children (diluted, of course) that can be used to calm irritable babies and toddlers and soothes temper tantrums. Roman chamomile oil is known for its amazing anti-inflammatory properties. It is widely used for soothing inflamed skin. Not just that, it also offers a natural solution for arthritis, muscle pain, sprains and persistent headaches.

16. Black Pepper Oil

The aroma of black pepper essential oil will often remind you of fresh ground pepper in the kitchen, with some floral and forest notes. It has a fundamental benefit over peppercorns. Unlike black peppercorns, it does not make you sneeze or cause irritation to the senses. You may not use it on its own, but it can be used brilliantly to add more spice to the blend as a middle note that's neither too heavy nor too light. Black pepper oil is versatile and can blend well with most floral, spice and citrus based notes.

Medically, black pepper essential oil helps facilitate blood circulation, reduces pain and tension in the muscles and can be an effective natural remedy for arthritis.

On the emotional level, black pepper essential oil acts as a stimulator and energizer. It is known to boost alertness and energy. For this reason, it is best avoided before going to bed. It is generally considered great for boosting stamina and can be used by athletes for that added energy zing.

17. Lime Oil

Lime essential oil is one of the most affordable and goodness-packed essential oil that is utilized for energizing the senses, spreading an aroma of freshness, cleaning a space and making the environment more positive and cheerful. Traditionally, lime oil was known for its cleansing, rejuvenating and purifying properties. It was known to renew and refresh the body, mind and spirit. Spiritually, lime oil is used for aura cleansing.

The fragrance of lime is sweet yet citrusy, which is what makes it a highly versatile blend oil. The aroma of concentrated lime essential oil can be very powerful and long-lasting. Blend it with different oils to create a citrusy blend for the diffuser to cleanse and purify rooms. You can also use lime essential oil for creating natural, homemade room mists that smell awesome without weighing heavily on the pocketbook.

18. Grapefruit Oil

Grapefruit oil has a nice, pleasant, sour and sweet fragrance that makes it a must-have versatile essential oil in the house. Owing to its sweet and tart nature, it blends effortlessly with several essential oils. You can blend it with frankincense and fir essential oils for a woody, earthy fragrance.

Apart from being wonderfully fragrant, grapefruit is also extremely energizing without being too strong. When you need as hot of energy or positivity (especially before heading to work or starting your daily chores in the morning), try diffusing it around the home. Combine it with other energizing and stimulating oils such as rosemary to add a sweeter note to the blend.

List of Essential Oils and Their Benefits

Here is a handy list of essential oils and their basic uses if you are just getting started with them. Though every essential oil can be used in a variety of ways depending on your creativity and resourcefulness, these are their general or most common benefits. The list is not in any particular order.

Cinnamon – Ensures oral hygiene and health, boosts metabolism, alleviates menstrual problems

Cedarwood – Excellent insect repellent, good for skin, keeps you emotionally upbeat

Black Pepper – Good anti-oxidant and blood circulation facilitator

Cardamom – Boosts digestion and tackles respiratory issues

Basil – Excellent for menstruation issues, helps combat sore muscles and ensures mental alertness and focus.

Chamomile – Boosts overall immunity, calms the mind and body

Cassia – Boosts the body's digestive functions and acts as a sexual stimulant

Cilantro – Enhances digestive processes, purifies blood, gives glowing skin and is a natural anti-oxidant

Arborvitae – Good for cleansing and an effective insect repellent

Clary Sage – Balances hormones effectively, alleviates stress and tension, good for maintaining emotional balance and an effective agent for tackling PMS elated issues.

Clove – Ensures oral health, boosts immunity and is good for the heart.

Lemongrass – Induces a calming feel, boosts digestion, great for the complexion and excellent insect repellent

Marjoram – Good for heart health, offers muscle support and helps maintain emotional balance

Lime – Boosts energy and stimulates, great detoxification agent and improves overall functioning of the immune system

Myrrh – Good for the skin, effective cleansing agent and helps maintain emotional balance

Oregano – Effective cleansing agent, helps the digestive system and good for fighting respiratory issues

Rosemary – Effective against respiratory disorders, boosts memory, good for digestion and improves hair and scalp health

Orange – Provides emotional balance, excellent purifying and detoxification agent and acts as an energizing stimulant

Peppermint – Excellent cooling agent, offers an energy boost, effective for digestion and fights respiratory ailments

Frankincense – Great for emotional and mental balance as well as glowing skin

Lavender – Versatile essential oil used for stress and anxiety relief, fighting persistent headaches and keeping the skin healthy

Grapefruit – Stimulating and energizing agent, ensures alertness of mental faculties, great cleansing remedy, ensures skin health and suppresses appetite

Jasmine – Effectively balances moods and emotions and ensures skin health

Eucalyptus – Acts as a good cleaning agent, combats respiratory problems and offers healthy, glowing skin

Cypress – Energizes, boosts skin health and alleviates muscle tension

Tea Tree – Superb cleansing agent, ensures skin health and boosts overall immunity

Sandalwood – Calming agent, effective against stress and anxiety and effective grounding agent

Thyme – Excellent insect repellent, effective for cleansing and purification purposes and boosts overall functioning of the immune system

Spearmint – Effective against bad breath, ensures oral health and good for the digestive system

Tangerine – Energizing agent, good for cleansing and purification and boosts overall immune system

Ylang-Ylang – Excellent calming agent and ensures glowing hair and skin health

Bergamot – Ensures emotional and mental balance, great mood booster, and combats skin problems effectively

Fennel – Ensures effective blood circulation, facilitates metabolism and boosts overall digestion

Wintergreen – Ensures emotional balance, offers relief against sore muscles and gives glowing skin

Patchouli – Offers healthy skin, effective tension and stress reliever and great grounding agent

Geranium – Effective insect repellent, calms nerves and improves skin and hair condition

Thyme – Great for cleansing and purifying, boosts the immune system and is a proven insect repellent

Fir – Good for fighting respiratory conditions, relaxes tense muscles and reduces joint pain

Conclusion

Thank you for downloading *Essential Oils: A Practical Guide for Beginners*.

I genuinely hope you enjoyed reading this book. I also hope the book has given you lots of practical, quick, resourceful and effective ideas for getting started with essential oils.

There's just no limit to what can be done with essential oils, and the number of ways in which you can include it in your daily life to enjoy its benefits in the area of home, health and beauty.

The next thing to do after reading this beginner's handbook of essential oils is to use all the tips, ideas and recipes mentioned. Do not just read. Apply what you learned. By using essential oils, you will notice greater balance in your physical and mental state.

Lastly, if you enjoyed reading the book, please take the time to share your thoughts by posting a review on Amazon. Your feedback is greatly appreciated.

Here's to transforming your home and health with the goodness of essential oils!

Works Cited

Barnes, P M, E Powell-Griner, K McFann, and R L Nahin. 2004. "Complementary and alternative medicine use among adults: United States, 2002." *Advance Data* (343): 1-19.

Lee, K B, E Cho, and Y S Kang. 2014. "Changes in 5-hydroxytryptamine and cortisol plasma levels in menopausal women after inhalation of clary sage oil." *Phytotherapy Research* 1599 - 1605.

Naik, M I, B A Fomda, E Jaykumar, and J A Bhat. 2010. "Antibacterial activity of lemongrass (Cymbopogon citratus) oil against some selected pathogenic bacterias." *Asian Pacific Journal of Tropical Medicine* 3 (7): 535 - 538.

PDQ Integrative, Alternative, and Complementary Therapies Editorial Board. 2005. *Aromatherapy and Essential Oils (PDQ®)*. Review, National Cancer Institute, Bethesda: PubMed Health. Accessed October 11, 2017. https://www.ncbi.nlm.nih.gov/pubmedhealth/PMH0032645/.